I0757098

Lose Belly Fat Burn Undesired Fats Now

MAHDJOUBI ZINEDDINE

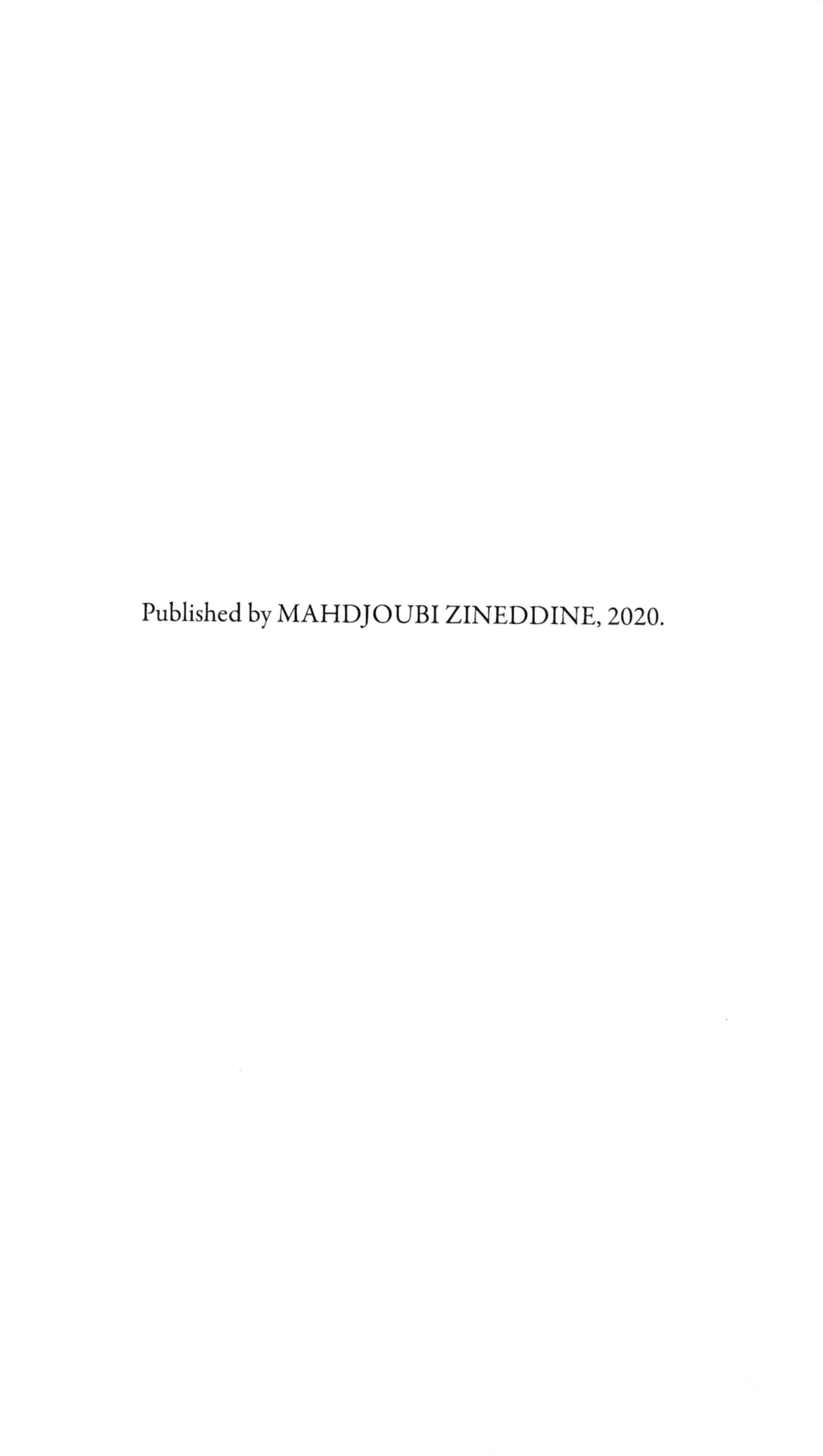

Published by MAHDJOUBI ZINEDDINE, 2020.

While every precaution has been taken in the preparation of this book, the publisher assumes no responsibility for errors or omissions, or for damages resulting from the use of the information contained herein.

LOSE BELLY FAT BURN UNDESIRED FATS NOW

First edition. September 3, 2020.

Copyright © 2020 MAHDJOUBI ZINEDDINE.

Written by MAHDJOUBI ZINEDDINE.

God !

Thank you for giving me *life* , and *Honored* me
.To All people who i met and i meet in my life

Thank you for being a nice part of my life .

Chapter one : a General look at intermittent fasting

Hello and welcome .in this book we will learn about how to burn

Belly Fats like pro Star in the Spot light .we will burn fat and lose weight at 90/100 success at least and for that believe me you need to show us the beast that lives inside you , show the world how brave you are through your self Disciplin .

let us talk about Some basic topics , about what to do and what not to do , it is very simple but powerfull so focus and take notes to remember how and what to do easily .

let us start with this , begin with 3 meals and then go

to two you don't want to eat all day because every time you eat you spike

a hormone that prevents weight loss called insulin ,so eating in general generates a lot of insulin that fights to never make a fat burn this is why we fail at diet , because we eat and spike insulin that makes fats impossible to burn .

we don't want to do . Snacking againe and againe between meals going to create a big

problem for you so removing the snacking is vital .that is why we do

intermittent fasting. So here I suggest you start with three meals and then do that for a while get into ketosis or fat-burning and then

go to two meal. insulin is the hormone that is responsible for the

midsection weight so keep having only three meals with no snacking. You need also Protein so 100 gr to 200 gram per meal will help you and make you comfortable , but too much meat

will stimulate insulin be carefull .

next secret is eating 500 gr to 1 kg of veggies because we need to flesh out

all this fat that's going to be coming out to your liver all the fat through the body has to go through the liver and if you don't eat enough vegetables

you can cause fatty liver ,also vegetables give us the potassium . we need to

consume the vegetable first and have a big big big salad and then a small amount of

protein. Also we do not need sugar because sugar increases insulin

and also invisible sugars the breads pasta cereal cookies

biscuits pancakes muffins alcohol etc .. cut the sugar and

refined carbs out , now look at this secret ,healthy fats this is essential such as Olive OIL because when you consume fat at the end of the meal that allows you to go to the next meal

without being hungry in craving and starving that your blood Sugar's crash

so this basically allows you to do three meals or two meals without being hungry while not increasing insulin. Look at this magic FAT is one of the Beautyfull things that does not increase insulin it's neutral and safe .next secret is eating enough potassium why

because at the deep of weight loss we want to avoid insulin and so most people

that can't lose weight have too much insulin they suffer from insulin resistance so

we want to fix insulin resistance. potassium is a key , you can have it from vegetables or even from some other sources like supplements in order to fix dysfunction of insulin. Now we need apple cider vinegar because the acid in apple cider vinegar

does improve the output of insulin. it reduces insulin it improves insulin

resistance it lowers your blood sugars this is why it's very good for diabetics ,just take

in the morning one teaspoon with a glass of water and one before bed or

2 to 5 with your dinner if you have digestive issues.Also we need B vitamins especially vitamin b1 for

regulating insulin control and improving insulin resistance, you can use nutritional yeast for that purpose .now it is time to practice some sets and reps we need to workout with high-intensity interval training if you add high-intensity

when you make 30 Squats and rest for 15 second 10 times in your training you're gonna spike growth hormone and you're gonna speed up weight loss. the magic is making short periodes of high-intensity, and the most important thing is Sleeping ,and Recovery time

From doing high-intensity interval training

.now it is time to reduce stress ... believe me you have to live without stress because stress generates Cortisol and this is Bad because when cortisol is

triggered it will stop your weight loss and kills your efforts ,believe me you do not need that so evoid stress as hard as you can .and focus on doing your diet perfectly and Always remember : Perfect Performance leads to Perfect results ...

Chapter 2 : Reduce Stress ,now

All of our live we used to consume sugar as fuel to make cells work , then we try to Practice Intermittent Fasting to adapt our body to never use sugar as Fuel but to use Ketons as Fuel We Practice Intermittent Fasting to Generate Ketons Fuel from burning our Fats ..Look at this Champion , we burn Fats ,we Burn undesired Weight to Generate our Fuel and Energy source that Called Ketons ...but there is some mistakes you need to evoid ... focus with me on this topic : you lived a whole life eating huge Amount of carbohydrates your whole life ! ,now we'regoing to switch to ketones, so you're going to be adapted to the Ketosys Process wich is Generating Ketons through burning body fats such as Belly fats , if you're notbut to get Access to this Stage of Ketosys you need Time ,

LOSE BELLY FAT BURN UNDESIRED FATS NOW7

Time is Valuable thing , time is Key , some time is needed to adapt to this magical transformation of your body .At the very beginning you are consuming the sugar as fuel , your Body burns sugar that is Stored in your body , so you're just running on stored sugar which is called glycogen so it's stored in your muscles and your liver so when you go from one meal to the next over a period of time you're not switching to fat-burning if you're basically going to tap out your glycogen Reserve and the blood sugars are going to go lower .and when it goes lower it's going to activate adrenaline to raise it ,but in the process adrenaline is a stress hormone so it's going to activate the hypoglycemic symptoms and this is what happens with people making this transition into ketosis or they're adapting they get headaches , dry mouth and being thirsty theyget tired easy weak muscles craving irritable nervous all these symptoms so , and this is due to the Adrenaline that make a call to hormone , Cortisol will start increasing so we don't want to add that stress , because stress will lead to failure . this is WHY people Quit their diet and intermittent fasting plan , they work as hard as beasts ,they do every single detail with perfection But my friend STRESS kills their will , headache pains , weakness and being tired kills their dreams , but the reality it is not Pain who kills the process , Pain is a result of wrong acts 80/100 of time , when you feel pain you shall ask your self where is my wrong move in my diet plan , it may be that you eat too little food , or eat too much food , or bad timing , any thing it could be , you shall be Smart my friend .here's what you need to do you need to do it gradually so you start with three meals a day , with no snacking, do that until you're comfortable ,you can do iteasily. The Key of success here is , Do things **Gradually** ,then go three meals within an eight-hour period and a whole painfull 16hours of Hunger and starvation , then you go into two meals with an eight-hour period and a whole 16 hours of starvation time , it is achievable my friends , when you feel pain , your body is telling you show me your character , push through the pain , you must show self discipline , show your character , don't say why me but say come on Try me , at this point my friend you have done it , you have done it perfectly . now add some fat to the meal to go longer without feeling hungry when you Fast between meals , but go from 3 meals to 2 meals to 1 meal with gradual process , you need just some time a month or two to switch to fat-burning and you're running in your fat and you have no drop in blood sugars .so now let us pretend that you had two meals eight-hour period, now we're going to slowly go to seven hours of your window of eating , to have one meal seven hours later another meal then go six hours and then five and four , so you want to do it very gradually until you get comfortable so you don't have this adrenaline rush . because this is How you reduce stress , the key here is use your time , do not go quickly , play a long game not short game

and our game here is : **Pain and character** .

Chapter3 : What is intermittent fasting ?

Let us make things easy , visibly intermittent fasting is basically not eating so it's not starving
because you have time window of eating , look at this , people wanna know if they can have tea or coffee or supplements during the 16 hours of fasting , this is normal , have some tea or coffee without sugar of course , drink water when you want , yes you need some help , especially at morning , because almost at 8 oclock at morning when we wake up and get ready for school or work , body generates Cortisol , and cortisol causes stress , and we know that Stress is a Headache , stress is felling hungry , stress make things difficult , stress is Pain ..

this is where you have to discipline your behavior , and adapt your mind set to be beyonf pain , act smart , when you feel hungry and weak at morning get some tea to regulate your mood , believe me the pain will pass , you need just some time , you need just the self discipline and going through pain smartly . believe me the more you do this themore you're going to go from sugar burning to fat burning more efficiently that takes time though . so another factor is the estimation of effort it takes to really get into this hard core so you're fully in to keto where it'scomfortable you have cognitive benefits you feel focused you have concentration you have powerfull memory you can now learn faster so that's going to happen over time but for some people it could take three to four months. and I'm talking about weight loss too especially in your midsection , just push trough the pain and hunger and you will get your result you wil loose that weight . you will loose that belly fat . you will look beautyfull . just Push harder and Smarter .now imagine , you're doing all these multiple meals per day , it is now Hight time to do not eat Carbs like Pasta , bread , biscuits ....this is Key .the other Key is to add enough vegetables to also help you go from one meal to the next , the global mistake that people do it without enough vegetables ,you need vegetables for the potassium and magnesium and the other minerals and vitamins that help heal insulin resistance and help lower insulin as well as the fiber that feeds the microbes in your gut and that produces something called butyric acid and this helps insulin resistance it stops hunger it helps blood sugars it feeds the colon cells and i tenhances your immune system . the combination of good fat and vegetables is going to help you go from one step to the next and then just let your body dictate when to eat so you'regonna find you can go longer . so you can easily skip the breakfast now you're at two meals a day and now you start to act Smarter , use good fats like olive oil + enough vegetables ,let your body tell that champion now i am ready to go to next Level , i am adaptable to just having one unique meal per day .and take notes :you need this : 1 spoon of sea salt per day , body needs sodium .you need electolytes , you find it in lemon , make a lemon juice every day .milk , yogurt and bananas are rich of electrolytes also . you need electrolyte to enhance your muscle tissues and enhance your nerves and to feel energitic and evoid feeling weak and fatigue , so it is important .you need : vitamines and minerals you can find them in vegetables and fruites , but i'd rather having vitamins and minerals as supplements since they are available with low costs every where .you need also : vitamine B , you can find it at nutrution yeast or get it as supplement . it is available every where .you need to : never eat carbs that will give you maximum results , and makes you loose a huge amount of fat within short amount of time .you need to never eat sugar againe , because we do not need it , while adapting to the Ketosys stage ,you will feel better without eating sugareven is it seems hard at the begining .remember our fight is about : PAIN and Character .

Chapter4 : lose belly fat ,new overview.

Here we are going to lose that weight , here you are adapting with a new mindset , new concept of losing weight .

How many times people you know or heared about practicing inlimited amount of time with intermittent fasting and keto diet but they had no good results , no serious loss of weight .now , if they read this they will make it and they will lose that big fats , they will burn that numerous kilograms of fats . now all you need is this FOCUS and GO FORWARD .

Now look at this , we practice intermittent fasting and keto diet to get Healthy , right ! but we are wrong , we follow a wrong concept , we try hardly to lose weight in order to get healthy .

But the true concept and the logical way is to get healthy at the first place then lose weihts .... ! do you get the idea !

Why ? because your fats and weight is a symptom it's not the cause it's a Results of an

unhealthy body, so now losing weight is logicaly very unnatural to the body the body

doesn't like to lose weight at this moument , it fights against its purpose to survive, so it

doesn't lose like to lose anything so the weight is the tip of the iceberg.

the real Mindest and true Concept is something has to

do with a very specific hormone, that's holding down your metabolism ,there are

two sets of hormones hormones that make you gain weight and hormones that help

you lose weight, most global advice focuses on the calories while ignoring

the hormone triggers, instead they try to stimulate the metabolism they try to

give you an appetite suppressant they're trying to push you do some type of trick to trick your metabolism to some exercise or kinds of workouts but that is never going to work.because they follow a wrong concept and a wrong technics , it is always about science and logic

never break science and logic rules because i twill never work .

here at this point it is vital to know that the thing that stops and kills your weight loss process

is called insulin.it is something weird but it is true ,

a lot of people think that this Hormone

concerns only diabetes but it has another function a magical function and it

is the hormone that puts fat not only on your body but mainly your midsection , are you taking notes champion , it focused mainly on your midsection it

also prevents you from losing weight it's called the fat storage hormone and

here's what people don't realize in the presence of even very little bit of

insulin all fat burning hormones are shut down.

Here my friend it is : GAME OVER .

what does that mean it means

Insulin is up = you gain , insulin down=you lose weights .

When you see someone big be sure that he has a lot of insulin in his body .

The question is what can i do to make insulin down ?

One of magic question is :

A low-carb diet , when you cut out carbs believe me you are on the right path to lose weight .

Cuting carbs out is Healthy . keep in mind that sugar is your enemy even if it is Sweet . it is a Smooth criminal . Dangerous , when you eat sugar be sure that some bad things are watching you lol .cut out sugar , carbs , hidden sugar like pasta and muffins , potato , rice ... ride on the right plane to fly to the successfull results .now take a look at this Magical secrets i challenge you if you heared about befor in Media or newstv ..

One magical secret that people don't realize, that low fat proteins trigger insulin more than fattier proteins.do you follow me ! Low fat protein makes you fattier meanwhile fattier proteins makes you lose weights ... magic , right lol.

Look at this , when you eat at restaurants delicious food and tasty meats , you shall know that those products contains monoglutamate it is a kind of Salt , they add to make food tasty and delicious .

But the bad thing is it double the insuline amount 200/100 so next day you feel that you gained inch or two of fats .... !

At this Point it is important to take a look at

insulin resistance condition , insulin acts like a key in the cells to open a door for nutrition that fuel the cells , but too much insulin is bad , body resist it and changes the doors locks , so insulin as a key can not open the new locks , now we are in trouble .

people with insulin resistance have five

to seven times more insulin than normal people

so if you were to test someone of insulin resistance they might have

normal blood glucose but they have very high insulin levels. This is a real Fact , but the doctors

never check that you would have to test a fasting insulin test not a fasting

glucose test completely different right and insulin
resistance is the

pre-diabetic State but a lot of times it will not show
up on normal tests until

it's too late. And you become a diabetic. so now let
me show you the

symptoms of insulin resistance .

number one belly fat despite how many sit-ups or
crunches

you do you cannot lose your belly fat no matter
what.

number two you get plateaued

just by eating healthy. number three when you eat
carbohydrates you feel better it

reduces your stress you become less cranky and before you crave sugar and

carbs number five a need for a nap and want to sleep after lunch believe me this is a Key sign of insulin resistance .

number six brain fog dementia absent-mindedness you start lacking the

clarity of focus especially when you don't eat .

number seven worse eyesight

especially as the day progresses it's like you're at night your vision is

worse .look at this , diabetic they go blind why because the

blood sugars are needed to be normalized to actually feed the eye so since in

some resistance is the pre-diabetic State

you could have vision problems well before diabetes . and it's just bad

eyesight next one not satisfied after you eat you know you need a little

something sweet after you'll eat why because the cells are insulin resistance they're blocking insulin and so you can't get the fuel in the cell so the

cells are starving yet you gain only this way you become fatter yet you're

starving to death.oh my god ! may god helps us . are you focusing friend ! when you need sweets after eating it is because nutrition are not getting into cells because cells resist insulin that try to open the doors locks . so cells are starving , they get zero fuel and they make zero energy while nutrition is stored as fats due to that huge amount of insulin .. this is powerfull and very worst thing can happen,wich god help us and protect us from this things .

next one the need to urinate

the middle of the night wherever the sugar goes the water goes so in other

words you might have fluid retention but you also might be just peeing in the

night once or more than once and that is a process symptom of a pre-diabetic symptom of insulin resistance number 10

swollen belly as the day progresses do you find that in the morning your

stomach is a little bit lower but at in the day it's swole up or maybe you have

to eat it just swells up that's insulin resistance so you can see insulin

creates a lot of problems now there are also danger-ous long-term side effects of

too much insulin as well heart disease, diabetes as you might already know a

fatty liver ,high blood pressure is too much insulin that's why when you actually fix the in-sulin issue the blood

pressure comes down ,high cholesterol because in-sulin converts sugar into

cholesterol and triglycerides stroke has been con-nected to high levels of insulin

dementia is little plaquing in the brain that stops the brain from working and

Alzheimer's amyloid plaques it's called that comes from too much insulin so you

can see that insulin is the common denominator for so many health problems

that go beyond just belly fat .so let us be more responsible and give our selves and our kids the right food and helthy way to live with .

our fight Here is : Beyond the weight loss

Chapter 6 : now , read and lose weight right here .

In this part you will lose the most inwanted weight , you will burn the Maximum fats ,you will burn as much fats as you want , Here in this chapter , you will work hard and show your self discipline , just understand my words and practice what i am saying to you , and you lose weight all the weight that you do not want will be burnt , now .but i ask from you just one thing my friend , i Ask you to show free will and self discipline through courage and going forword beyond pain ... that is what it takes

.carbs : you want to lose Fats and fat weight , you do not want to lose muscles , or lose just water weights , so take this :1/ Stop eating **carbs Now.** You will get some carbs when eating vegetables , but it is ok , i want you to get Healthy during this diet plan , So let carbs be as close to zero ,and this will give you huge results and impressive weight loss .Look at this , while someone practice diet plan , sometimes it do not work , because of something called insulin resistance it is a problem when your body does not use insulin while producing huge amount of it , so insulin protect fats from being Burnt as Fuel !so we have must to Regulate that insulin resistance 2/ eat 1.5 Kg of green vegetablesand salads .this is a Super magical secret maybe 90/100 of people who want to lose weight do not event know about it !!Let me explain

something funy : though vegetables gives us energy and

vitamins and minerals , but the funny thing , we want

to feed our colon microbs with those vegetables ! weird

thing , is'nt it ?This is the fact that you don't read at

school , whenhealthy microbes eats vegetables , theyg ive

as in exchange something called Butyrate .Butyrate is

more valuable than gold , believe me , butyrate controls

our insulin rates, it restore the original normal insulin

rate at blood , so all of that huge amount of insulin will

disapear ...Insulin will act normaly with normal amount

. and when insulin is down to the normal , Results will

be Beautyfull , weight loss will be the most effective that

you can get .This is when magic happens ...... it is just about butyrate ...so , Eat vegetables champion and re-store your beautyfull body back .

/3Protein and fats

In this stage , we need Protein to help our muscles to get repaired at the time they need this ,

You need to eat 100 grams per meal , if you are big or you do intermittent fasting plan with 1 or two meals per day , you may want to add more protein but the max-imum is 200 grams per meal .

Also you need healthy fats to consume with the meat you eat bcause fat reduces amount of insulin , because when you eat meat you spike insulin , and fats you eat re-duce that insulin and keep your weight loss process safe .

You can eat different kind of meats , i do not recom-mend pork meats , because it is very dirty , porks eats any thing and that affects its meat , you can eat beef meat or any meat you want, fish , salmon or sardines are rich of omega-3 and other important elements that body needs and even our brain needs .

Eggs are very good , you can consume 2 eggs per meal .

Whe it comes to fats , i like to take fatty meat with some fats , animal fats or olive oil is good .it is easy to understand : meat+fats= safe weight loss process .

Chapter 7 :How to kill cancer and generates new stem cells , generate new brain cells , kill viruses ......

Look at this Honey , let us get more Healthy , let us kill all kinds of Cancers , repeat with me :

Here we kill cancer , and this is how we do .

Honey , imagine a tumer of Cancer is in someone body , maybe in his leg or even orse in his Head...

Focus with me honey , when we practice fasting for long times such us 48 hours ...

Of course we drink water and take nutrition minerals and vitamins ... the point is fasting for 48 hours and keep rising the periode ... what will you get in exchange ... is something called Autoimmune condition or what we call the Blessed stage of Autophagy ...

Autophagy , is a condition where your body eats maximum of your fats and feels like this is not enough for him , so Body start eating viruses , microbes and can-cers ... at the end of the day , a virus is a combination of proteins , a cancer is a combination of proteins that is charger to destroy your cells

, so honey , take this , Cancer is surviving through eating your Blood sugar ... Cancers eats Only Sugar ... this is it is point of strenght , But infact it is Cancer's biggest Point of weak ...

How is that , Cancer grow and grow hile eating your sugar , cancers are addicted to sugar , this is why doctors test for cancers bygiving a person flueressent sugar , and they follow where that Sugar is going the most ... it must go somewhere with huge weird amounts ... sugar must go to Cancer tumeurs ,

But what is killing cancer is the fact that cancers can never eat Ketons , it can not eat Ketons as a fuel , so when you start fasting for 2 days and more , your body enters the stage of Ketosys , your body burns your fats to feed it self while there is no glucose in blood , there is only ketons to fuel only the body .. At this point Cancers are hungry and Starving , they feel tired and get worst condition ever . they can no longer resist immune system , cancer now is very weak , almost like huge numbers of enemy soldiers , but these soldiers are starving and being hungry since months , now these soldiers are very skinny and weak , Fatigue killing them , they can no longer fight or even run or lift something heavy , they just begging for food , this is where our soldiers our immune system kills all these enemy once for all .. believe me it is a massacre , a war crime , but this war Crimes keeps Human race living more and more , it gives us hope , it heel us , and erases our Pain ...

Immune system now destroy those cancers and viruses and the funny thing body start to urn them into fuel and ketons .. and get the bad elements like heavy metals or bad things out of body ....

How great is our Body ...

I try to make the idea as easy as i can to show you the way that our body works .. man ! we are great , we are beautyfull ! i admit that the God creator that creates human being is more greater and is the most beautyfull !!

God creator , we love you , keep raise on us and help us more and more , and guide us to know you more and more . thank you god .

Remember :

1/Start intermittent fasting with 3meals

2/move to 2 meals only after you get used to intermittent fasting

3/eat 2 kilograms of greens and salads , use what you can find in market .

4/eat 100 grams to 200 grams of protein each meal then reduce it one by one

5/eat 50 grams to 100 of healthy fats i recommend extra virgin olive oil or fats that comes with sheep meats

6/Fats reduces your insulin amount ,and makes you feel no hunger any more so you can stand between your meals .

7/never take snacks between meals

8/cut Sugar and hidden Sugar out .

9/Cut the carbs now .

10/take menerals multiple and multy vitamines p, c ,d ,b ....buy it as supplements

11/if you feel you need to eat Bread take vitamine B . all kind of vitamine b is recommended

12/consume electrolytes , make lemon juice in you 16 hours of intermittent fasting , you find also electrolytes in Banana fruits wich i recommend for you the most with lemons , also milk contains it .

13/never eat pork meat because it contains a lot ofmicrobes in its blood and that affects its meat ..

14/feel what your body is saying , feel your pain and head aches , resist pain smartly , when you feel hunger killing you it is a sign that you are burning fats now , when you feel hunger pain while you are fasting , make some coffee or thea with no sugar added , never use nescafe it is not good for fasting .

15/drink 4 liters of waterevery day , you need water to burn that fats .

16/show your self discipline , strugle is beautyfull , it is a sign of your success , remember pain is temporarly thing , it will pass , keep fasting and keep going forword , winners walk on , go forword with the best mindset , walk through pain and get your goal .. Lose weight now .

17/while planing to reduce stress and reduce Cortisol amounts especially at 8 oclock , at morning , make your coffee , feel blessed, and love your family , kiss your kidsand feel happy .

18/ last tip is : Put god first .. God creates us to live healthy and happy , and he gave us the power of commitment and discipline to achieve our goals , you know Sky does not rain gold nor silver , we need to work hard to live ... think about it , rain , is a result of days of days of work from the sun light to vaporise sea water , then wind collect it in the sky as a cloud form , then it travels across the world to rain at the end of the trip at a faraway place ... this is what i call Power of Time ... go with your plan nice and easy ... use time .. we have a lot of time but every second counts .

Win the long game and the result will be impressive ....

So , when i look at the whole process , i thank god who gave me brave and courage to achieve my goal and lose my weight and burn my belly fat wisely ...

Honey , this is the end of the trip with me seeking for weight burning , thank you for reading my words and keep in mind : i love you honey .

Don't miss out!

Visit the website below and you can sign up to receive emails whenever MAHDJOUBI ZINEDDINE publishes a new book. There's no charge and no obligation.

https://books2read.com/r/B-A-USVL-DPNIB

BOOKS 2 READ

Connecting independent readers to independent writers.

www.ingramcontent.com/pod-product-compliance
Lightning Source LLC
Chambersburg PA
CBHW040309240726
48664CB00006B/1439